SHIATSU FOR BEGINNERS

Comprehensive Guide To Massage Techniques, Pressure Points, And Self-Care Practices For Effective Stress Relief And Wellness

DR SAWYER DIEGO

TABLE OF CONTENTS

CHAPTER ONE 11

SHIATSU OVERVIEW 11

ORIGIN OF SHIATSU 11

SHIATSU TRAINING'S HEALTH AND WELL-BEING ADVANTAGES.......12

KNOWING THE FUNDAMENTALS OF SHIATSU'S ENERGY FLOW 14

FUNDAMENTAL ANATOMY CONCEPTS RELATED TO SHIATSU..........15

ORGANIZING YOUR AREA FOR SHIATSU EXERCISE.....................17

CHAPTER TWO 19

FUNDAMENTALS OF SHIATSU 19

OVERVIEW OF JAPANESE MASSAGE TECHNIQUES KNOWN AS SHIATSU..19

AN UNDERSTANDING OF ACUPRESSURE POINTS AND 20

SHIATSU TECHNIQUES FOR APPLYING PRESSURE' 22

THE VALUE OF AWARENESS AND RELAXATION IN SHIATSU 24

FUNDAMENTALS OF SHIATSU'S YIN AND YANG.........................26

CHAPTER THREE 29

GETTING READY FOR A SHIATSU TREATMENT 29

ESTABLISHING A RELAXED SETTING FOR SHIATSU 29

CLOTHES OBSERVATIONS FOR THE PRACTITIONER AND CLIENT 30

EQUIPMENT AND TOOLS REQUIRED FOR SHIATSU PRACTICE 32

SAFETY MEASURES AND PERSONAL HYGIENE.........................33

PERFORMING AN ASSESSMENT AND INTAKE OF CLIENTS 35

CHAPTER FOUR 37

FUNDAMENTAL SHIATSU METHODS...37

OVERVIEW OF TECHNIQUES FOR FINGER AND PALM PRESSURE 37

SHIATSU JOINT MOBILIZATION AND STRETCHING TECHNIQUES 39

PRESSING INTO CERTAIN ACUPRESSURE POINTS 40

INCLUDING RELAXATION BREATHING TECHNIQUES 42

CHANGING PRESSURE BASED ON CUSTOMER INPUT 43

CHAPTER FIVE 45

SHIATSU FOR TYPICAL HEALTH ISSUES 45

APPLYING SHIATSU TO REDUCE STRESS AND PROMOTE RELAXATION
.... 45

USING SHIATSU TO TREAT HEADACHES AND MIGRAINES 46

METHODS FOR RELAXING THE SHOULDERS AND NECK 48

ENHANCING THE QUALITY OF SLEEP WITH SHIATSU 49

CONTROLLING ANXIETY AND ENCOURAGING EMOTIONAL 50

CHAPTER SIX 53

USING SHIATSU TO BALANCE ENERGY 53

COMPREHENDING THE SHIATSU IDEA OF ENERGY IMBALANCE 53

METHODS FOR USING SHIATSU TO BALANCE QI 54

USING SHIATSU TO BOOST GENERAL VITALITY AND ENERGY 56

CONSISTENT SHIATSU PRACTICE IS ESSENTIAL FOR 58

CASE STUDIES HIGHLIGHTING SHIATSU'S BENEFICIAL EFFECTS 59

CHAPTER SEVEN 61

ADVANCED METHODS OF SHIATSU 61

SHIATSU'S DEEP TISSUE TECHNIQUES 61

SHIATSU METHODS FOR PARTICULAR SITUATIONS 62

INCLUDING JOINT ROTATIONS AND PASSIVE STRETCHING 64

SHIATSU IN COMBINATION WITH OTHER COMPLEMENTARY 65

SHIATSU SESSIONS CUSTOMIZED FOR EACH CLIENT 67

CHAPTER EIGHT..69

INCLUDING SHIATSU IN EVERYDAY LIFE..69

SELF-SHIATSU METHODS FOR PERSONAL WELLNESS 69

SHIATSU EXERCISES TO PRESERVE YOUR MOBILITY AND 70

INCLUDING SHIATSU IN A HOLISTIC HEALTH PRACTICE 72

INCLUDING SHIATSU IN YOUR MEDITATION AND YOGA 73

REGULAR SHIATSU PRACTICE HAS LONG-TERM HEALTH 75

CHAPTER NINE 77

PROFESSIONALISM AND ETHICS IN SHIATSU PRACTICE.........................77

THE VALUE OF MORAL PRINCIPLES IN SHIATSU...............................77

PRESERVING THE PRIVACY AND CONFIDENTIALITY OF CLIENTS 78

SETTING PROFESSIONAL LIMITS IN THE PRACTICE OF SHIATSU........80

SHIATSU PRACTITIONERS' PROFESSIONAL DEVELOPMENT AND 82

LEGAL ASPECTS AND RULES APPLIED TO SHIATSU PRACTICE 83

CHAPTER TEN 87

GETTING STARTED IN SHIATSU 87

HOW TO ACQUIRE CERTIFICATION AS A SHIATSU PRACTITIONER.....87

ESTABLISHING A SHIATSU PRACTICE: SITE AND SUPPLIES 88

MARKETING TECHNIQUES TO DRAW CUSTOMERS TO YOUR 90

STRATEGIES FOR RETAINING CLIENTS AND DEVELOPING A..............92

BUDGETING AND FINANCIAL ISSUES FOR A SHIATSU PRACTICE........93

CHAPTER ELEVEN 95

SHIATSU FAQS AND TROUBLESHOOTING 95

RESOLVING FREQUENTLY ASKED QUESTIONS ABOUT LEARNING SHIATSU...95

FAQS REGARDING SHIATSU METHODS AND THEIR USES...................96

SOLVING CLIENT PROBLEMS IN SHIATSU SESSIONS............................98

HOW TO TAKE CARE OF YOURSELF AND AVOID BEING A 100

RESOURCES FOR CONTINUING EDUCATION AND CAREER...............101

ABOUT THE BOOK

"Shiatsu for Beginners" is a thorough guide for anyone interested in learning more about the traditional Chinese medicine-based Japanese massage therapy known as "Shiatsu," Shiatsu emphasizes the manipulation of meridians and acupressure points to enhance the body's inherent healing abilities and restore balance. The book starts by examining the fundamentals of Shiatsu, outlining its historical foundations, and outlining how it enhances general health and well-being.

A key component of Shiatsu practice is an understanding of the flow of energy, or Qi, which gives practitioners insights into how to rebalance energy for optimal health.

Shiatsu-related anatomy is also covered, guaranteeing a strong basis for practice. Finally, practical advice on creating a comfortable and relaxing environment for Shiatsu sessions guarantees relaxation and comfort for both client and practitioner.

The fundamentals of Shiatsu massage are thoroughly examined, providing an outline of the different methods that are employed to apply pressure on particular points along the body's meridians. Methods include joint mobilization, stretching, and pressure with the fingers and palms, all of which are intended to relieve tension in the neck and shoulders, reduce stress, and enhance emotional and physical health.

Integrative approaches combine Shiatsu with complementary therapies like yoga and meditation, enhancing its therapeutic benefits. Advanced techniques go deeper into tissue manipulation and specific applications for conditions like back pain and digestive issues. Professional boundaries and confidentiality are two ethical considerations unique to Shiatsu practice, ensuring practitioners maintain high standards of care and respect.

With resources for continued learning and development, "Shiatsu for Beginners" is more than just a guide—it's a gateway to embracing Shiatsu as a holistic approach to health and healing. FAQs address common concerns and troubleshooting tips ensure practitioners are equipped to handle various client needs effectively. For those who aspire to become Shiatsu practitioners, this book offers a roadmap for certification, practice establishment, marketing strategies, and client relationships.

CHAPTER ONE

SHIATSU OVERVIEW

ORIGIN OF SHIATSU

The term "shiatsu" means "finger pressure" in Japanese, referring to the emphasis on applying pressure with the fingers, thumbs, and palms to specific body points to facilitate healing and balance. Shiatsu originated from traditional Chinese medicine and Japanese massage techniques, specifically Anma, and incorporates ideas from acupuncture and acupressure.

Based on the theories of traditional Chinese medicine, which emphasizes the balance of energy (Qi) within the body, Shiatsu originated in Japan in the early 20th century.

One of the key figures in the history of Shiatsu is Tokujiro Namikoshi, who established the first Shiatsu clinic in Japan in 1925 and was instrumental in formalizing the practice by focusing on anatomical understanding and helping to establish Shiatsu's legitimacy within the Japanese medical community.

Shiatsu is now practiced all over the world, with practitioners having modified and improved its techniques to meet the demands of modern practice. Although it still has its traditional roots, modern Shiatsu incorporates a deeper understanding of human anatomy and physiology, making it a flexible and successful therapy for a range of health conditions.

SHIATSU TRAINING'S HEALTH AND WELL-BEING ADVANTAGES

Learning Shiatsu has many advantages for both physical and mental health. Stress reduction and relaxation are two of the main benefits.

The firm but gentle pressure used in Shiatsu sessions calms the nervous system, releases tension from the muscles, and promotes deep relaxation, which can enhance sleep, lessen anxiety, and increase overall well-being.

Regular Shiatsu practice can help maintain flexibility and mobility, making it beneficial for those with musculoskeletal issues or sedentary lifestyles. Shiatsu also improves circulation and stimulates the body's natural healing processes. By targeting specific points along the body's meridians, or energy pathways, Shiatsu can improve blood flow, increase lymphatic drainage, and boost the immune system. This can help alleviate chronic pain, reduce inflammation, and support recovery from injuries.

Beyond its physical benefits, Shiatsu is beneficial for mental and emotional well-being. The practice's holistic approach recognizes the body, mind, and spirit as interconnected.

By promoting inner harmony and balancing the body's energy flow, Shiatsu can help release emotional blockages and improve mental clarity as well as emotional resilience and life's ability to handle challenges.

KNOWING THE FUNDAMENTALS OF SHIATSU'S ENERGY FLOW (QI)

Qi, the life force that permeates the body, is central to Shiatsu. In traditional Chinese medicine, Qi circulates along certain pathways called meridians. The body is healthy and balanced when Qi flows freely; blockages or imbalances in Qi can result in physical, emotional, and mental health problems. Shiatsu works to restore the proper flow of Qi, thereby promoting overall well-being.

In addition to using their hands, fingers, and palms to apply pressure to specific points along the meridians—which correspond to different organs and systems within the body—Shiatsu practitioners also use joint rotations, stretches, and gentle manipulations to support the free movement of Qi. By stimulating these points, Shiatsu practitioners help to release blockages, enhance energy flow, and restore balance.

One of the main tenets of Shiatsu is that physical symptoms can be caused by energy imbalances. For instance, pain or tension in a specific area may be a sign of a blockage in the corresponding meridian. Through knowledge of and work with the body's energy pathways, Shiatsu practitioners can treat the underlying causes of health problems instead of just treating their symptoms, ensuring a thorough and long-lasting healing process.

FUNDAMENTAL ANATOMY CONCEPTS RELATED TO SHIATSU

Fundamental knowledge of anatomy is essential for practicing Shiatsu effectively. Practitioners can apply safe and accurate pressure by knowing about the skeletal, muscular, and nervous systems. The spine, joints, and major muscle groups are important anatomical structures for Shiatsu because these areas are frequently the focus of treatment.

Since the spine supports the body's structure and houses the spinal cord, it is a key component of

Shiatsu. Practitioners can treat conditions like tension headaches, sciatica, and back pain by understanding the vertebrae and the nerve pathways that connect them. They can also perform safe and effective stretches and manipulations by knowing how the spine aligns and moves.

Shiatsu practitioners benefit from an understanding of muscle anatomy because many of the techniques involve applying pressure to particular muscle groups to release tension and enhance circulation. Knowing the major muscles, such as the deltoids, hamstrings, and trapezius, allows practitioners to target these areas with effectiveness. Additionally, knowing the functions of muscle attachment points helps practitioners address muscular imbalances and promote overall flexibility and strength.

Finally, understanding the nervous system is essential to understanding how Shiatsu works on the body. The nervous system regulates the movements and sensations of the muscles, and pressure applied to specific points can either stimulate or calm nerve activity. By knowing this, practitioners can adjust their techniques to achieve specific therapeutic goals, such as relaxation or pain relief.

ORGANIZING YOUR AREA FOR SHIATSU EXERCISE

Shiatsu requires a specific space for both the practitioner and the recipient. To promote healing and relaxation, the space should be quiet, comfortable, and distraction-free. To start, pick a quiet room where you have control over the lighting and temperature. Ambient lighting and a comfortable temperature help to create a calming atmosphere that promotes relaxation.

A comfortable mat or futon for the recipient to lie on should be provided by the treatment area; the mat should be supportive but not too firm; there should be enough room surrounding the mat so that you can move freely and apply pressure from different angles; and necessary supplies like pillows, blankets, and towels should be easily accessible to support the recipient's comfort and positioning during the session.

An inviting and well-kept space not only makes the recipient feel at ease but also frees you up to concentrate on providing an efficient and thoughtful Shiatsu treatment. Regularly clean the mat and any equipment to ensure a hygienic environment. Arrange your tools and materials neatly. Consider adding elements that enhance the ambiance, like calming music, essential oil diffusers, or plants.

CHAPTER TWO

FUNDAMENTALS OF SHIATSU

OVERVIEW OF JAPANESE MASSAGE TECHNIQUES KNOWN AS SHIATSU

Translating as "finger pressure," shiatsu is a traditional Japanese massage therapy in which pressure is applied to specific body points to balance the body's energy, or "qi," to promote relaxation, reduce stress, and improve overall health. Shiatsu practitioners apply pressure along the body's meridians or pathways through which energy flows, with their thumbs, fingers, palms, and occasionally even their elbows and knees. The ultimate goal of shiatsu is to remove blockages and restore the natural flow of energy, thereby enhancing the body's inherent healing capabilities.

In a typical Shiatsu session, the client remains fully clothed while the practitioner observes and palpates the client's body to determine which areas require attention and how much pressure to apply.

The practitioner may utilize a variety of techniques, including gentle stretching, tapping, and rotating limbs, in addition to applying pressure. Because each session is customized to the client's specific needs, Shiatsu is considered a highly personalized form of therapy.

Shiatsu has many health benefits, such as relieving chronic pain, strengthening the immune system, improving circulation, increasing flexibility, and improving emotional and mental well-being by lowering anxiety and depression. Shiatsu also supports overall health and wellness by promoting the flow of qi and restoring balance within the body, making it a valuable practice for anyone looking to improve their physical and emotional well-being.

AN UNDERSTANDING OF ACUPRESSURE POINTS AND MERIDIANS

The body's energy flows through invisible channels called meridians; in Shiatsu, knowledge of these channels is essential because it helps the practitioner determine where to apply pressure. There are twelve main meridians, each of which are linked to a particular organ and represent a different aspect of emotional and physical health; for example, the lung meridian is associated with grief and respiratory health, while the liver meridian is linked to anger and detoxification. By working along these channels, practitioners hope to balance the body's energy and facilitate healing.

Acupressure points, also called tsubo, are particular places on the meridians where energy tends to concentrate. These points can get blocked or imbalanced because of a variety of things, like stress, poor diet, or inactivity. Acupressure practitioners can release blockages and restore the flow of energy by applying pressure to these points; each point has a specific function and can affect different body parts. For example, applying pressure to the Hegu point on the hand can help relieve headaches, while stimulating the Zusanli point on the leg can improve digestion and bolster the immune system.

To effectively treat clients, a practitioner of Shiatsu must have a thorough understanding of the body's energy pathways and how to manipulate them to achieve desired results. This understanding enables the practitioner to create targeted treatments that address the underlying causes of a client's symptoms rather than just treating the symptoms themselves. Shiatsu places a strong emphasis on the holistic health of the individual, to bring about long-lasting improvements in both physical and emotional well-being.

SHIATSU TECHNIQUES FOR APPLYING PRESSURE'

Shiatsu requires more than just applying pressure to the body; to provide effective treatment, the practitioner must understand how to use their body weight, posture, and alignment. One of the basic techniques is the use of the practitioner's thumb, which is frequently used to apply concentrated, deep pressure to particular acupressure points. The thumb should be firm but relaxed, and the practitioner should use their body weight rather than just their muscle strength to exert pressure. This ensures a consistent, penetrating pressure that can effectively stimulate the body's energy flow.

Beyond the thumb, Shiatsu practitioners apply pressure with their fingers, palms, elbows, and even their knees; each provides a unique quality of touch and can be used to achieve a variety of therapeutic effects. For example, the palm is frequently used for broader, more diffuse pressure, which can help relax larger muscle groups and promote a general sense of relaxation; fingers and elbows can provide more concentrated pressure, which is ideal for working on specific points or smaller areas of tension; knees and forearms can be used for deep, sustained pressure, especially on larger muscle groups like the back and thighs.

To apply pressure correctly, one must also be aware of the direction and rhythm of the application; pressure should be applied gradually, building to the desired intensity and then released slowly; this prevents pain or discomfort and allows the body's energy to adapt to the stimulation; practitioners frequently move in a fluid, continuous manner, following the body's natural contours and the meridians' flow; this rhythmic, mindful application of pressure not only enhances the therapeutic effects but also promotes the client's general relaxation and well-being.

THE VALUE OF AWARENESS AND RELAXATION IN SHIATSU PRACTICE

Both the client and the practitioner benefit greatly from relaxation and mindfulness in Shiatsu. The practitioner can apply pressure with precision and sensitivity when they are fully aware of the client's needs and can adjust their technique based on the client's feedback and responses. The practitioner can also benefit from mindfulness by maintaining proper body mechanics and posture, which lowers the risk of strain or injury and increases the effectiveness of the treatment.

To fully benefit from Shiatsu, the client needs to relax; a relaxed body is more responsive to the therapeutic effects of pressure and manipulation; additionally, relaxed bodies allow the body's energy to flow more freely, which facilitates the release of tension and the restoration of balance; clients are frequently encouraged to practice mindfulness during sessions, which helps to deepen the state of relaxation and fosters a sense of peace and well-being.

Shiatsu emphasizes relaxation and mindfulness, which not only addresses physical ailments but also supports emotional and mental well-being, contributing to a holistic sense of health and balance. Adding mindfulness to Shiatsu practice can also improve the relationship between the practitioner and the client, which is crucial for effective healing. The practitioner's mindful presence and the client's relaxed state create a harmonious environment where the body's natural healing processes can be activated.

FUNDAMENTALS OF SHIATSU'S YIN AND YANG

Yin and Yang, which have their roots in traditional Chinese medicine, symbolize the dualistic nature of all things in the universe. Yin is connected to attributes like darkness, coolness, passivity, and receptivity, while Yang is associated with qualities like light, warmth, activity, and dynamism. In the context of Shiatsu, these principles aid practitioners in comprehending the flow and balance of energy within the body. They also help practitioners understand how illness or discomfort develops when this balance is upset.

Practically speaking, Yin and Yang dictate how techniques are applied and what the focus of treatment is in Shiatsu. For example, a condition with excess Yang, like tension or inflammation, might be treated with calming, cooling techniques that enhance Yin qualities; on the other hand, a condition with excess Yin, like sluggishness or coldness, might be treated with stimulating, warming techniques that boost Yang energy. Practitioners can customize their approach to help clients regain harmony and balance in their bodies by understanding the nature of their conditions in terms of Yin and Yang.

Comprehending Yin and Yang also facilitates practitioners' work with the body's meridians more effectively. Based on location and function, meridians related to the lower body and internal organs are typically more Yin, whereas meridians related to the upper body and external functions are more Yang. This categorization guides practitioners' approach to different parts of the body during treatment. Shiatsu seeks to balance the Yin and Yang energies within the meridians to address the physical as well as the emotional and mental aspects of the patient's ailment.

CHAPTER THREE

GETTING READY FOR A SHIATSU TREATMENT

ESTABLISHING A RELAXED SETTING FOR SHIATSU

For a Shiatsu session to be successful, the client and the practitioner must be in a calm and peaceful environment. To start, choose a quiet area that is free from noise and distractions. Soft lighting can help promote relaxation; think about using candles or dimmable lights to create a calming atmosphere. Natural light can also be helpful, as long as it is not too harsh. To further enhance the calmness, play soft, ambient music or nature sounds in the background. This auditory element can help drown out any leftover noise and promote relaxation.

A futon or massage table with a supportive mat and pillows should be available to ensure the client is comfortable and properly supported throughout the session. Additionally, consider adding elements like plants or aromatherapy diffusers with calming scents like lavender or chamomile to enhance the overall peaceful ambiance of the room. Make sure the temperature of the room is comfortable, adjusting the heating or air conditioning as necessary. A space that is too cold or too hot can distract from the session.

Personal belongings should be put away, and any equipment that is not in use should be neatly arranged. This helps create a professional and serene space that helps the client feel at ease and ready to receive the full benefits of Shiatsu. Maintain the space clean and uncluttered because a tidy environment promotes a sense of order and tranquility.

CLOTHES OBSERVATIONS FOR THE PRACTITIONER AND CLIENT

Wearing loose, comfortable clothing made of natural fabrics, such as cotton, allows the practitioner to apply pressure and manipulate the body without restriction. Tight, restrictive clothing, or anything with too many zippers and buttons, can help prevent discomfort and interfere with the treatment. Proper clothing is important for both the client and the practitioner to ensure comfort and ease of movement during a Shiatsu session.

Equally important is the practitioner's attire, which should be comfortable, flexible, and allow for a full range of motion. Simple, professional clothing would be yoga pants or loose-fitting trousers paired with a simple top; this allows the practitioner to move freely around the client and apply various techniques without restriction. Simple, non-slip footwear would be clean, flat shoes that provide stability or socks with grip.

By following these clothing guidelines, both the client and the practitioner can ensure a smooth and effective Shiatsu session. Strong perfumes and lotions can be distracting and may interfere with the session. Jewelry should also be kept to a minimum to prevent any accidental discomfort or damage.

EQUIPMENT AND TOOLS REQUIRED FOR SHIATSU PRACTICE

A comfortable futon or massage table is essential as it provides a stable and supportive surface for the client to lie on; this should be paired with pillows and bolsters to support different body parts, ensuring maximum comfort and proper alignment throughout the treatment. Although the tools and equipment needed for Shiatsu practice are relatively minimal, each piece plays an important role in ensuring a successful session.

Practitioners may also use small towels to cover specific areas of the body, providing modesty and comfort for the client during the session. Finally, a lightweight blanket can be useful for keeping the client warm and comfortable. Clean, soft towels or sheets are necessary to cover the futon or table, maintaining hygiene and providing a pleasant surface for the client to lie on. These should be changed after each session to ensure cleanliness.

Shiatsu is primarily performed with the hands of the practitioner; however, some practitioners may augment the treatment with acupressure balls or small wooden implements, which can help apply more precise pressure to specific body points.

The most crucial "tool" in Shiatsu is still the practitioner's skilled touch, which means that a thorough understanding of the body's meridians and pressure points is essential.

SAFETY MEASURES AND PERSONAL HYGIENE

To protect both the client and the practitioner, safety, and hygiene are crucial in Shiatsu practice. To start, make sure the treatment area is sanitized and clean; all linens, including sheets, towels, and pillowcases, should be laundered between sessions; and the practitioner washes their hands thoroughly before and after each treatment to maintain a high standard of hygiene and prevent the spread of germs.

Clear communication is essential; practitioners should regularly check in with clients to ensure that the techniques and pressure being used are comfortable and effective. Throughout the session, the practitioner should be aware of the client's comfort and any potential contraindications. It is imperative to avoid applying pressure to areas where the client has reported pain, injury, or discomfort unless specifically trained to address such conditions.

In addition, to give the best care possible, practitioners should maintain their physical well-being. This includes using proper body mechanics to prevent strain and injury while performing Shiatsu techniques; keeping nails clipped; and avoiding overly strong fragrances or lotions; by following these safety and hygiene guidelines, practitioners can create a clean, safe, and effective environment for Shiatsu therapy.

PERFORMING AN ASSESSMENT AND INTAKE OF CLIENTS

The first steps in getting ready for a Shiatsu session are a thorough client intake and assessment. Have the client fill out an intake form that covers their medical history, current health conditions, and any specific concerns or goals they may have for the session. This will help the practitioner better understand the client's overall health and customize the treatment to meet their needs.

To get more in-depth information from the client during the first consultation, have a thorough conversation with them. Ask open-ended questions about their lifestyle, stress levels, and any physical or emotional issues they may be dealing with. These kinds of dialogue helps establish rapport and trust, which helps the client feel more at ease and ensures that the practitioner has a thorough understanding of their needs. Taking note of the client's posture, gait, and breathing patterns can also yield important information about their physical state.

A comprehensive intake and assessment allows practitioners to ensure that each Shiatsu session is customized to provide the client with the maximum therapeutic benefit. Based on the information gathered, the practitioner can create a personalized treatment plan that addresses the client's specific needs and goals. This plan should be flexible, allowing for adjustments based on the client's response during the session.

CHAPTER FOUR

FUNDAMENTAL SHIATSU METHODS

OVERVIEW OF TECHNIQUES FOR FINGER AND PALM PRESSURE

Shiatsu practitioners apply pressure to specific body points using their thumbs, fingers, and palms. The first step in applying pressure is placing the thumb or finger on the targeted area and pressing steadily and evenly.

The pressure should be firm but not painful, and it's crucial to keep your posture relaxed to prevent tension from being transferred to the client. By using your body weight instead of just your muscle strength, you can apply pressure to a deeper, more effective treatment.

Practicing palm pressure regularly helps to develop the sensitivity needed to gauge the appropriate pressure for different body parts. Palm pressure techniques involve using the entire palm to cover larger areas of the body, such as the back or thighs. To apply palm pressure, place the palm flat against the skin and lean in with your body weight, allowing the pressure to sink deeply into the tissues. This method is particularly useful for relieving tension in large muscle groups and promoting overall relaxation.

The goal is to promote healing and relaxation, so always make sure the client is comfortable and receptive to the treatment.

To increase the effectiveness of finger and palm pressure, practice mindfulness pay attention to changes in muscle tension, and adjust your pressure accordingly.

These techniques, when combined with slow, deliberate movements, help to achieve a harmonious flow, which facilitates better energy circulation throughout the body.

SHIATSU JOINT MOBILIZATION AND STRETCHING TECHNIQUES

Joint mobilization and stretching are essential elements of Shiatsu that work to increase joint health and flexibility. To work on a limb or joint, support it gently. For example, hold the elbow and wrist while slowly extending the arm to its full length. Apply light pressure to encourage a deeper stretch. Make sure the movements are controlled and smooth to avoid pain or injury.

Joint mobilization is a technique that helps improve circulation around the joint and release tension by gently moving the joint through its range of motion. For example, when working on the shoulder, support the client's arm and move it in circular motions, gradually increasing the range as the joint loosens.

It is important to communicate with the client throughout the process and modify the intensity of the mobilization or stretch based on their feedback.

Stretching and joint mobilization combined with pressure techniques help to address both muscular and joint issues, offering a comprehensive treatment; regular practice and attention to the client's responses ensure these techniques are performed safely and effectively, contributing to overall physical well-being. Including these techniques in a Shiatsu session can greatly increase the therapeutic effects.

PRESSING INTO CERTAIN ACUPRESSURE POINTS

To facilitate healing and energy flow, Shiatsu therapy targets specific acupressure points. To apply pressure to these points, locate the area using anatomical landmarks and traditional Chinese medicine charts. Once the point has been identified, use your thumb, finger, or knuckle to apply firm, steady pressure. The duration of the pressure application varies, ranging from a few seconds to a minute, depending on the sensitivity of the point and the comfort level of the client.

Some common acupressure points are those on the hands, feet, and along the spine. Each point corresponds to different organs and systems in the body, so learning their locations and functions is crucial for effective treatment. Acupressure point pressure can vary, so for beginners, it's important to start with moderate pressure and gradually increase it as needed. Make sure the pressure is consistent and avoid abrupt changes in intensity.

Your ability to provide targeted relief will improve with regular practice and familiarity with acupressure points. You can also create a more holistic treatment approach by learning about the meridian system and how these points are connected.

You should always watch the client's reaction and modify the pressure accordingly to ensure a therapeutic experience that is both balanced and supportive of general health and well-being.

INCLUDING RELAXATION BREATHING TECHNIQUES

Encourage clients to take slow, deep breaths during the session to help release tension and promote a sense of calm. Teach them to inhale deeply through the nose, filling the lungs, and then exhale slowly through the mouth. This rhythmic breathing pattern helps synchronize the body's energy flow with the therapeutic pressure applied. Breathing techniques are a powerful addition to Shiatsu therapy, enhancing relaxation and the overall effectiveness of the treatment.

Exhaling as you apply pressure and inhaling as you release is a technique that not only improves your well-being but also fosters a more harmonious energy exchange between you and the client. As a practitioner, your breathing is equally important. You can provide more effective treatment by keeping a steady, deep breathing pattern that helps you stay focused and calm.

During the session, remind the client to pay attention to their breath, particularly during periods of intense pressure or stretching. This mindful approach to breathing not only helps with relaxation but also amplifies the therapeutic benefits of Shiatsu, which will have a more profound and long-lasting effect on the client's overall health. Guided breathing exercises can be incorporated into the session to further enhance relaxation.

CHANGING PRESSURE BASED ON CUSTOMER INPUT

For a Shiatsu treatment to be both safe and effective, pressure must be adjusted in response to feedback from the client. Discuss comfort levels and any specific areas of concern at the beginning of each session. Throughout the treatment, keep lines of communication open by asking the client to let you know if the pressure is too light or too intense. This way, the treatment will be customized to meet their unique needs and preferences.

Develop a rapport and trust with the client so that they feel more comfortable providing honest feedback. Pay close attention to non-verbal cues like changes in breathing, muscle tension, and facial expressions.

These indicators can provide valuable information about the client's comfort level even if they don't verbally communicate it. If you notice signs of discomfort, adjust the pressure immediately and follow up with the client to make sure the new intensity is appropriate.

Incorporating client feedback into your technique not only improves treatment efficacy but also cultivates a more positive and cooperative experience. Your ability to be attentive and responsive helps to establish trust and create a more comfortable environment for the client. This way, every session is tailored to the individual needs of the client, maximizing the therapeutic benefits of Shiatsu and promoting long-term wellness.

CHAPTER FIVE

SHIATSU FOR TYPICAL HEALTH ISSUES

APPLYING SHIATSU TO REDUCE STRESS AND PROMOTE RELAXATION

Using your thumbs to apply steady pressure in circular motions, gently press and knead the shoulder and neck areas to release tension that has built up in these common stress-holding areas. Work slowly, focusing on your breath, and encourage the recipient to do the same, creating a calming rhythm that enhances relaxation. Shiatsu can be a very effective method for relieving stress and promoting relaxation.

Then work your way back, using your palms to apply firm, consistent pressure along the spine; adjust the pressure according to the recipient's feedback. As you work, gently rock to release any tightness in the muscles and create a calming, peaceful atmosphere. This rhythmic motion helps to reduce stress because it relaxes the muscles and calms the nervous system.

At the end of the session, both the giver and the receiver should noticeably feel less stressed and more at ease. The hands and feet are often neglected but can hold a lot of tension. To help release blocked energy and promote deep relaxation, use your thumbs to press into the reflex points, starting from the base of the hand or foot and working towards the fingertips or toes.

USING SHIATSU TO TREAT HEADACHES AND MIGRAINES

Shiatsu is a helpful technique for treating headaches and migraines. Move in small, circular motions, breathing deeply and encouraging the recipient to do the same, as this helps relax the muscles and reduce headache intensity.

Start by concentrating on the head and neck areas, as these are often the sources of headache pain. Use your fingertips to apply gentle pressure on the temples, gradually increasing the intensity to a comfortable level.

Then, focus on the base of the skull and the upper neck. Press firmly and steadily with your thumbs on either side of the spine, working slowly outward from the center. This technique targets the occipital points, which can greatly relieve tension headaches and migraines. Hold this position for a few minutes, keeping your rhythm steady to help release tight muscles and enhance blood flow.

For all-encompassing relief, concentrate on the hands and feet as well. For the hands, target the big toe by pressing and holding the area just below the toenail, which can help alleviate migraine symptoms. These techniques, when combined, can provide effective relief from headaches and migraines.

Press into the webbing between the thumb and index finger, a well-known acupressure point for headache relief. Apply firm pressure for about one minute, then release and repeat on the other hand.

METHODS FOR RELAXING THE SHOULDERS AND NECK

Effective methods for releasing tension in the neck and shoulders include: having the recipient lie down or sit comfortably; starting with the shoulders, working from the neck outward to the arm, and using your thumbs to apply firm downward pressure, which helps release the built-up tension that often builds up in this area. Use kneading motions and vary the pressure to ensure a deep, therapeutic effect.

Next, work on the neck. Cradle the recipient's head gently in your hands, then apply pressure with your thumbs along the sides of the neck, working from the base of the skull down to the shoulders. While you're at it, gently tilt the head to each side and hold it there for a few breaths before releasing it. This will help to lengthen the neck muscles, which will improve flexibility and reduce stiffness.

Lastly, concentrate on the upper back. With the patient on their stomach, apply firm, sweeping pressure from the center of the back out towards the shoulders. Include rocking motions to further release the muscles and encourage relaxation.

The space between the shoulder blades is a common location where tension accumulates. These Shiatsu techniques can greatly reduce tension in the neck and shoulders, offering both short-term and long-term relief.

ENHANCING THE QUALITY OF SLEEP WITH SHIATSU

Starting the session with light pressure on the scalp, and using your fingertips to massage the head in slow, circular motions, can help to calm the mind and prepare the body for deeper relaxation. Encourage the recipient to focus on their breathing, taking slow, deep breaths to enhance the soothing effects. Shiatsu can greatly improve the quality of sleep by promoting relaxation and reducing stress.

Next, work on the feet. Press firmly into the soles, kneading and pressing in circular motions with your thumbs. Concentrate on the arches and heels, which are important areas for relaxation. This helps to ground the recipient and activates the reflex points that support general relaxation and well-being. Work on each foot for several minutes, making sure to cover it completely to achieve the most calming effects.

The recipient should feel deeply relaxed and prepared for a restful night's sleep by the end of the session. The last area to work on is the back and shoulders. With the recipient lying comfortably, use your palms to apply broad, sweeping pressure along the spine, from the lower back up to the shoulders. Include gentle rocking and stretching to further ease muscle tension. Pay particular attention to the areas around the shoulder blades and neck, as releasing tension here can significantly improve comfort and ease.

CONTROLLING ANXIETY AND ENCOURAGING EMOTIONAL HEALTH

Beginning the session with light pressure on the chest and abdomen, apply slow, rhythmic movements with your palms to help calm the heart rate and encourage deep breathing, both of which are important for reducing anxiety.

Encourage the recipient to focus on their breath, taking slow, deep inhalations and exhalations to enhance the calming effect. Shiatsu is a useful tool for managing anxiety and promoting emotional well-being.

Next, work on the hands and arms. Press firmly along the meridians with your thumbs, from the wrist to the elbow. This releases trapped energy and encourages harmony and balance. Work on each arm for several minutes, making sure to cover all the areas. This helps to ease tension in the body as well as to release emotions, which helps with anxiety management.

Incorporate gentle stretches by tilting the head to each side, and holding the position for a few breaths before releasing it. This helps to release tension and promote relaxation. Lastly, work on the neck and shoulders.

Using your fingertips, gently press along the sides of the neck, moving down to the shoulders. By the end of the session, the recipient should noticeably feel less anxious and more emotionally balanced.

CHAPTER SIX

USING SHIATSU TO BALANCE ENERGY

COMPREHENDING THE SHIATSU IDEA OF ENERGY IMBALANCE

Energy, or Qi in traditional Chinese medicine, flows through specific pathways in the body called meridians; when Qi flows freely, the body is in a state of balance and health; however, if Qi flow is disrupted due to stress, poor diet, or lack of exercise, it can result in physical and emotional imbalances, which can manifest as symptoms like fatigue, anxiety, or chronic pain, indicating that certain areas of the body are either deficient or excessive in energy. This concept is fundamental to Shiatsu's understanding of how the body works and how to restore health.

A Shiatsu practitioner will perform a comprehensive assessment to find energy imbalances; this may involve palpating the meridians and observing the client's posture, skin condition, and breathing patterns, among other things. The practitioner's objective is to find areas where Qi is stagnant or blocked and ascertain the underlying causes of these disruptions. By identifying the specific patterns of energy imbalance, practitioners can customize their treatments to meet each client's individual needs, guaranteeing that the therapy is both effective and holistic.

To correct energy imbalances, methods are used to bring the body's natural energy balance back. Shiatsu, for example, uses light pressure and specific meridians to manipulate points to clear energy pathways and allow Qi to flow freely throughout the body. This process not only relieves symptoms but also supports general health by re-establishing the body's natural energy balance.

METHODS FOR USING SHIATSU TO BALANCE QI

In Shiatsu, balancing Qi is achieved through a range of techniques that concentrate on different aspects of the meridians and pressure points. One basic technique is the application of pressure to specific acupoints along the meridians using the thumbs, fingers, palms, or elbows; this stimulates the flow of Qi, aiding in the release of blockages and the restoration of balance; the amount of pressure applied can vary from gentle to firm, depending on the sensitivity of the client and the condition being treated.

To further open up the meridians and improve the flow of energy, stretching is another essential technique. It can be done in two ways: passively, in which the practitioner moves the client's limbs into different positions, or actively, in which the client participates by moving or holding certain postures. Stretching not only improves flexibility but also permits a deeper release of tension and a more profound regulation of Qi.

To address energy imbalances, Shiatsu practitioners also use joint mobilizations and rotations. By gently rotating and moving the joints, they can help to release stagnant Qi and encourage a more even distribution of energy throughout the body. These techniques work especially well for areas that are prone to tension and stiffness, like the neck, shoulders, and lower back, offering relief and improving overall feelings of relaxation and well-being.

USING SHIATSU TO BOOST GENERAL VITALITY AND ENERGY

Targeting specific energy points and meridians, shiatsu encourages the body's self-healing mechanisms, helping to prevent illness and maintain optimal health. Shiatsu is well known for its ability to enhance overall energy and vitality by promoting the free flow of Qi throughout the body. Regular shiatsu sessions can help to invigorate the body's natural energy reserves, leading to increased stamina, mental clarity, and emotional balance.

Shiatsu promotes vitality through a variety of means, including improved circulation.

Shiatsu's rhythmic pressure and movements encourage lymphatic drainage and blood flow, both of which are vital for cell nutrition and toxin removal. Better circulation also improves the oxygenation of tissues and organs, which raises energy levels and supports the body's overall functioning.

Additionally, Shiatsu has a profound effect on the nervous system. The treatment's calming and balancing effects help to reduce stress and anxiety, which are common energy drainers.

Shiatsu's holistic approach not only addresses physical symptoms but also supports emotional and mental health, making it a powerful tool for enhancing overall vitality and energy.

 By encouraging relaxation and a sense of peace, Shiatsu allows the body to recharge and rejuvenate, leading to a greater sense of vitality and well-being.

CONSISTENT SHIATSU PRACTICE IS ESSENTIAL FOR MAINTAINING ENERGY

Consistent Shiatsu sessions support the harmonious flow of Qi in the body and help prevent the accumulation of energy blockages and imbalances that can cause illness and fatigue, keeping the body in a state of equilibrium. Regular Shiatsu practice is essential for maintaining energy balance and general health, much as physical fitness can be achieved through exercise and a healthy diet.

Weekly or biweekly Shiatsu can offer long-term benefits by continuously addressing and correcting minor imbalances before they become more serious problems.

This preventive approach to health care keeps the body's energy systems operating at peak efficiency, which fosters resilience and increased stress tolerance. Frequent Shiatsu practice also strengthens the immune system, which helps the body fight off infections and diseases.

In addition to being a time for relaxation and introspection, Shiatsu practitioners' regular sessions can help people become more aware of their bodies and their energy. Better lifestyle choices, such as regular exercise, a healthier diet, and stress-reduction tactics, can help people maintain their overall health and energy balance.

CASE STUDIES HIGHLIGHTING SHIATSU'S BENEFICIAL EFFECTS

Several case studies demonstrate how effective Shiatsu is at restoring energy balance and addressing a range of health issues. In one case, a middle-aged woman with anxiety and chronic fatigue reported significant improvements in her energy levels and a reduction in her anxiety symptoms following a series of Shiatsu sessions that addressed balancing Qi and relieving tension in the shoulders and neck. The practitioner employed a combination of pressure techniques and gentle stretching to encourage relaxation and unblock stagnant Qi.

Another case study involves a young athlete who was frequently suffering from fatigue and muscle strains. The athlete recovered more quickly and performed better after receiving regular Shiatsu treatments, which included deep pressure on particular acupoints and joint mobilizations. The targeted treatment helped to improve flexibility, release tension in the muscles, and increase overall vitality, demonstrating the benefits of Shiatsu for supporting physical health and athletic performance.

These case studies demonstrate how Shiatsu can effectively address a wide range of health issues by balancing Qi and supporting the body's natural healing processes. A third case study centers on an elderly man who suffers from arthritis and chronic pain. He finds that gentle pressure, stretching, and joint mobilizations during Shiatsu sessions significantly reduce his pain levels and improve his mobility.

CHAPTER SEVEN

ADVANCED METHODS OF SHIATSU

SHIATSU'S DEEP TISSUE TECHNIQUES

By carefully applying pressure on specific points along the body's meridians, practitioners of deep tissue Shiatsu work to release chronic tension and pain by targeting the deeper layers of muscle and connective tissue.

This technique requires a thorough understanding of anatomy and the ability to gauge the appropriate pressure for each individual, ensuring that it is both effective and comfortable. Deep tissue Shiatsu also helps to promote relaxation by releasing tight muscles and improving blood flow.

Deep tissue Shiatsu involves using techniques like kneading, rolling, and sustained pressure, with the practitioner continuously checking in with the client to ensure the pressure is tolerable. The goal is to break down adhesions in the muscle fibers and fascia, which can contribute to pain and restricted movement. The practitioner starts by warming up the area with lighter pressure, gradually increasing intensity to reach deeper layers. This is done slowly and deliberately to avoid causing pain or discomfort.

Deep tissue techniques are frequently used in conjunction with other Shiatsu techniques in a typical session to address the client's overall well-being. The practitioner may concentrate on particular areas of chronic tension, like the shoulders, back, or legs, and apply deeper pressure where necessary. This method, which promotes emotional release and mental clarity in addition to relieving physical discomfort, is an example of a holistic therapy that addresses multiple aspects of health.

SHIATSU METHODS FOR PARTICULAR SITUATIONS

Techniques such as gentle pressing, tapping, and stretching to relieve pressure on the vertebrae and surrounding muscles can be used by shiatsu practitioners to address a variety of conditions, including back pain, digestive problems, and more. For back pain, practitioners concentrate on key points along the spine and related meridians to release tension and improve alignment. This helps to reduce pain and improve mobility, offering both short-term and long-term benefits.

Shiatsu practitioners can help with digestive problems by applying techniques that stimulate the abdominal area and corresponding meridians. To improve bowel movements, reduce bloating, and enhance overall digestive function, gentle pressure is applied to points that influence digestion, such as the lower back and the Hara (abdomen). Techniques may include circular motions, gentle pressing, and rhythmic tapping to encourage the flow of energy and blood to the digestive organs.

Shiatsu can help alleviate the symptoms of headaches and migraines by focusing on specific points on the head, neck, and shoulders that are known to relieve tension and promote relaxation.

Overall, the practitioner's ability to customize techniques for specific conditions makes Shiatsu a versatile and effective therapy for a wide range of health issues.

INCLUDING JOINT ROTATIONS AND PASSIVE STRETCHING

Adding joint rotations and passive stretching to a Shiatsu session improves the client's range of motion and flexibility. Passive stretching is a technique where the therapist gently stretches the client's muscles without the client having to actively participate. It helps the client's muscles become longer, less stiff, and more mobile. People who are recovering from injuries or have limited mobility benefit most from passive stretching.

As an example, the practitioner might gently rotate the client's shoulders, hips, or ankles, paying close attention to any areas of restriction or discomfort. By methodically working through the joints, the practitioner can help to enhance the client's mobility and ease of movement. Joint rotations involve the practitioner moving the client's joints through their natural range of motion. This technique helps to lubricate the joints, reduce stiffness, and improve overall joint health.

In a Shiatsu session, these techniques are frequently incorporated to supplement other techniques and offer a more comprehensive treatment. For example, the practitioner may perform passive stretching and joint rotations to further enhance relaxation and mobility after applying pressure to specific points to release tension. This holistic approach guarantees that the client's body is balanced, flexible, and free of unnecessary tension, which contributes to their overall well-being.

SHIATSU IN COMBINATION WITH OTHER COMPLEMENTARY MEDICINES

Shiatsu can be used in conjunction with other complementary therapies to improve overall effectiveness and offer a more comprehensive approach to health and wellness. For instance, combining Shiatsu with acupuncture can help address the energetic as well as the physical aspects of a client's condition, as acupuncture uses fine needles to stimulate specific points while Shiatsu relies on manual pressure and meridians for its work.

The application of essential oils during a Shiatsu session can address particular health concerns and promote relaxation; for example, lavender oil can be used to promote calmness and reduce anxiety, while peppermint oil can invigorate and help with digestive issues. The combination of touch and scent creates a multi-sensory experience that can deepen the client's relaxation and overall therapeutic benefit. Aromatherapy is another complementary therapy that works well with Shiatsu.

Together with meditation, yoga, and shiatsu, clients can cultivate mindfulness, reduce stress, and maintain flexibility and strength in between sessions. By combining these complementary practices with shiatsu, clients can achieve a more harmonious and balanced state of health that addresses their mental and physical well-being.

SHIATSU SESSIONS CUSTOMIZED FOR EACH CLIENT

Shiatsu sessions must be tailored to each client's specific needs and preferences, which mean that each session must start with a thorough assessment in which the practitioner discusses the client's health history, current concerns, and specific treatment goals. This allows the practitioner to address the client's specific issues, such as chronic pain, stress, or digestive problems, in a way that is specific to them.

In the course of a session, the practitioner modifies techniques in response to the client's feedback and physical response. For instance, the practitioner may use lighter techniques or concentrate on different areas if the client feels uncomfortable with deep pressure; similarly, if the client has a specific condition, such as sciatica, the practitioner may use techniques that are most effective for that condition to concentrate on releasing tension in the lower back and legs.

By continually adapting and personalizing the approach, practitioners can provide a highly effective and satisfying Shiatsu experience that supports each client's unique journey toward health and wellness. Customizing each session guarantees that the client receives the most appropriate and beneficial treatment possible. It also fosters a stronger therapeutic relationship, as clients feel heard and understood.

CHAPTER EIGHT

INCLUDING SHIATSU IN EVERYDAY LIFE

SELF-SHIATSU METHODS FOR PERSONAL WELLNESS

Using your thumbs, fingers, and palms, apply firm but gentle pressure to various body points known as acupressure points. Starting with the head and neck, use circular motions to release tension and improve circulation. Moving on to your shoulders and arms, press and knead the muscles to relieve stress and increase flexibility. Self-Shiatsu techniques are a wonderful way to incorporate the benefits of this traditional Japanese therapy into your daily routine.

Proceed to work on your torso, focusing on the areas where many people hold tension: your abdomen and lower back. Apply pressure in small, circular motions using your knuckles to massage these areas. For your legs, begin at the thighs and work your way down to the calves and feet.

This will help to release tension in your muscles and improve blood flow and energy circulation. Throughout the process, remember to breathe deeply and slowly to increase relaxation and effectiveness.

Self-shiatsu can be an empowering tool to manage stress, reduce pain, and improve overall well-being. Lastly, practice these techniques regularly, ideally at the same time every day, to develop a consistent self-care routine. Over time, you'll become more attuned to your body's needs and more skilled at targeting specific areas that require attention.

SHIATSU EXERCISES TO PRESERVE YOUR MOBILITY AND FLEXIBILITY

Start with basic stretching exercises that target major muscle groups. Start with the neck and shoulders, gently tilting your head to the side and rolling your shoulders to release tension. Move on to the arms and torso, using slow, deliberate movements to stretch and elongate the muscles. Shiatsu exercises are designed to maintain and enhance your body's flexibility and mobility, making them an excellent addition to your daily routine.

For your lower body, work on stretches that lengthen the hamstrings, quads, and calves. Start with your feet shoulder-width apart, bend forward slowly, and reach for your toes. Hold the stretch for a few breaths, then return to an upright position. Repeat this movement, and add variations like side lunges and hip openers to increase the range of motion. Incorporate dynamic movements like gentle twists and bends to engage your core and improve spinal flexibility.

Finally, wrap up with strengthening and stretching exercises, such as yoga poses. The downward dog pose stretches the entire back of the body, and the cat-cow stretch is especially good for the spine. These regular exercises can help prevent stiffness, improve posture, and support general physical health. The key is to incorporate these Shiatsu exercises into your daily routine to maintain optimal flexibility and mobility.

INCLUDING SHIATSU IN A HOLISTIC HEALTH PRACTICE

To incorporate Shiatsu into a holistic health regimen, combine it with other wellness practices to create a well-rounded, balanced lifestyle. To begin, schedule regular sessions of Shiatsu, either with a practitioner or on your own, to address specific health issues and enhance your general well-being. Then, complement these sessions with other holistic practices like eating a well-balanced diet, getting regular exercise, and getting enough sleep.

To further maximize the benefits of Shiatsu, consider incorporating mindfulness practices into your daily routine. Activities like meditation, deep breathing, and mindfulness exercises can help you stay present and reduce stress. These practices complement Shiatsu by calming the mind and body and increasing your resilience to everyday stressors. You should also think about adopting a balanced diet rich in whole foods, as proper nutrition supports the body's natural healing processes and amplifies the effects of Shiatsu.

Last but not least, make self-care and relaxation a priority in your holistic health regimen. Shiatsu can be combined with gentle yoga, tai chi, or even a stroll in the park to enhance overall wellness and relaxation. This will help you develop a holistic approach to health that supports mental, emotional, and physical well-being.

INCLUDING SHIATSU IN YOUR MEDITATION AND YOGA PRACTICES

Shiatsu can be used to enhance the benefits of both meditation and yoga. To improve the effectiveness and enjoyment of your yoga practice, start your session with a few minutes of self-Shiatsu to warm up your muscles and prepare your body for movement. You can also apply light pressure to important acupressure points on your head, neck, and shoulders to release tension and improve energy flow.

Incorporating Shiatsu techniques into your yoga practice can help to deepen stretches, improve flexibility, and enhance the mind-body connection.

For instance, while holding a forward bend, gently press on the acupressure points along your legs to increase the stretch and promote relaxation. Similarly, in seated poses, use your thumbs to massage the pressure points on your feet to help ground and focus.

Use Shiatsu as a tool for relaxation and focus in your meditation practice. A powerful practice that supports physical, mental, and emotional well-being is created when you combine Shiatsu with yoga and meditation. Before starting your meditation, spend a few minutes applying gentle pressure to the acupressure points on your face and head.

This can help to calm the mind and prepare you for a deeper meditative state. During meditation, if you notice any tension or discomfort in your body, use Shiatsu techniques to address these areas, allowing you to maintain a comfortable and focused posture.

REGULAR SHIATSU PRACTICE HAS LONG-TERM HEALTH BENEFITS

Shiatsu is a valuable addition to your wellness routine because it has many long-term health benefits. First, it helps reduce stress by promoting relaxation and calming the nervous system, which can lessen the negative effects of chronic stress on the body. You can also experience improved mental clarity and lower anxiety levels by regularly incorporating Shiatsu into your routine.

Pain relief is another important advantage of Shiatsu. It can be especially helpful in treating chronic pain conditions like headaches, back pain, and joint problems.

Shiatsu uses gentle pressure and stretching techniques that help to improve circulation, release tension from muscles, and encourage the body's natural healing processes. Regular Shiatsu sessions can eventually result in less pain and increased mobility and function.

Shiatsu helps to support the body's natural defenses and improve overall health by promoting better circulation and energy flow. Regular sessions can also improve digestion, energy levels, and sleep quality, all of which contribute to a greater sense of well-being. By committing to regular Shiatsu practice, you can enjoy these long-term health benefits and improve your quality of life. Lastly, regular Shiatsu practice can boost your immune system and overall vitality.

CHAPTER NINE

PROFESSIONALISM AND ETHICS IN SHIATSU PRACTICE

THE VALUE OF MORAL PRINCIPLES IN SHIATSU

Honesty, integrity, and respect for human dignity are among the ethical standards that Shiatsu practitioners must uphold. These standards help practitioners make decisions that put their clients' health and safety first. For example, a Shiatsu practitioner must always obtain informed consent before beginning any treatment, explaining the methods and potential effects to ensure the client is fully aware of what to expect.

Recognizing the boundaries of one's expertise is another aspect of incorporating ethical standards. A Shiatsu practitioner should not try to diagnose or treat conditions outside of their scope of practice, and they should refer clients to the appropriate healthcare professionals when needed.

This keeps the practice's professional integrity intact and guarantees that clients receive the best care possible. By honoring these boundaries, practitioners show their dedication to moral principles and raise Shiatsu's standing as a holistic healing modality.

Shiatsu practitioners must be flexible and considerate to ensure that their practice is inclusive and respectful of each client's individual needs and preferences. This creates a safe and welcoming environment where clients can fully benefit from the therapeutic effects of Shiatsu. Being culturally sensitive and able to treat clients from diverse backgrounds with respect and understanding also falls under the category of ethical conduct in Shiatsu.

PRESERVING THE PRIVACY AND CONFIDENTIALITY OF CLIENTS

Shiatsu practitioners are required to keep all client information, including health histories and personal details, strictly confidential. This means not disclosing any information to third parties without the client's express consent unless there is a legal obligation to do so. Secure storage of records and data is also essential to protect client privacy. Upholding client confidentiality and privacy is crucial to Shiatsu practice because it fosters trust and supports a safe therapeutic environment.

Practitioners should assure clients that their information will be used exclusively to provide effective treatment and will not be shared without their permission. In practice, confidentiality starts with the initial consultation, where the practitioner gathers information about the client's health and well-being. This information should be discussed in a private setting to ensure that the client feels comfortable sharing sensitive details.

To protect confidentiality and privacy during sessions, clinicians should establish a safe and private treatment space. They should also make sure that physical boundaries are respected and soundproof the treatment area to prevent conversations from being overheard.

Finally, they should be considerate of the client's comfort, covering them appropriately and only exposing the areas of the body that are being treated. This considerate approach highlights the significance of confidentiality and privacy in developing a trusting therapeutic relationship.

SETTING PROFESSIONAL LIMITS IN THE PRACTICE OF SHIATSU

Establishing clear guidelines about the length and frequency of sessions helps manage client expectations and preserves the professional nature of the relationship. Developing professional boundaries is crucial for preserving a positive and productive practitioner-client relationship in Shiatsu practice. These boundaries help define the limits of the therapeutic relationship and guarantee that both parties understand their roles and responsibilities.

Maintaining a professional demeanor helps clients feel safe and respected, fostering a productive therapeutic environment.

Practitioners must also set emotional boundaries, ensuring that their interactions with clients remain professional and focused on the therapeutic goals. This involves being empathetic and supportive without becoming personally involved in the client's personal life. Practitioners should avoid sharing too much personal information or engaging in non-therapeutic interactions that could blur the lines of the professional relationship.

Because Shiatsu is a hands-on therapy, physical boundaries are especially important. Practitioners should always ask permission before touching any part of the client's body and explain the purpose of each touch or movement. This helps clients feel respected and at ease, knowing that their personal space and autonomy are being honored. Practitioners should also be aware of non-verbal cues and respond quickly to any indications of discomfort or hesitation from the client. Maintaining a professional and ethical Shiatsu practice requires clear communication and respect for physical boundaries.

SHIATSU PRACTITIONERS' PROFESSIONAL DEVELOPMENT AND ONGOING EDUCATION

To maintain high standards of practice and stay up to date with the most recent developments in the field, Shiatsu practitioners must commit to continuing education and professional development. Attending workshops, seminars, and advanced training courses are examples of opportunities for practitioners to learn new skills and expand their knowledge. This dedication to lifelong learning benefits the practitioner as well as the clients they serve; for example, mastering new techniques or comprehending recent research can lead to more creative and effective treatment approaches.

To ensure that practitioners remain competent and confident in their practice, they should regularly read relevant journals, attend conferences, and participate in professional organizations. Networking with peers and experts in the field offers valuable opportunities for knowledge sharing, new insights, and professional growth.

Staying up to date on the latest trends and developments in complementary and alternative medicine is another aspect of professional development.

In addition, obtaining professional certifications and credentials can help practitioners become more credible and improve their career prospects. A practitioner's expertise and adherence to high standards of practice are validated by many professional organizations, and by obtaining these certifications, practitioners show that they are committed to excellence and ethical practice, which can draw in more clients and build a solid reputation in the community. In summary, continuing education and professional development are crucial elements of a successful and ethical Shiatsu practice.

LEGAL ASPECTS AND RULES APPLIED TO SHIATSU PRACTICE

Shiatsu practitioners must be aware of and abide by local, state, and federal regulations governing the practice of Shiatsu. These regulations may include licensing requirements, scope of practice limitations, and standards for professional conduct. Comprehending and upholding these legal requirements helps protect both the practitioner and the client, fostering a safe and ethical practice environment. Legal considerations and regulations are crucial aspects of practicing Shiatsu, ensuring that practitioners operate within the boundaries of the law and uphold professional standards.

A license to practice Shiatsu is often obtained after passing a certification exam and finishing an approved training program. This guarantees that practitioners have the knowledge and abilities needed to treat patients safely and effectively.

Practitioners also need to be aware of any changes to legislation that may have an impact on their practice, such as new requirements for continuing education or updates to health and safety regulations. By routinely reviewing legal guidelines and consulting with legal counsel when needed, practitioners can better navigate the challenges of regulatory compliance.

In addition, legal considerations also entail knowing and putting into practice appropriate business practices, such as getting liability insurance and keeping accurate records. Liability insurance shields practitioners from lawsuits about their practice, giving them financial security and peace of mind. Accurate and thorough documentation of treatments and client interactions is crucial for legal compliance and can also be useful in the event of disputes or audits. Shiatsu practitioners can guarantee a respectable and long-lasting practice by following legal requirements and upholding professional standards.

CHAPTER TEN

GETTING STARTED IN SHIATSU

HOW TO ACQUIRE CERTIFICATION AS A SHIATSU PRACTITIONER

To become a certified Shiatsu practitioner, you must go through a series of organized steps to master this holistic healing art. To start, look for accredited Shiatsu training programs that fit your schedule and goals. Look for schools that are recognized by reputable Shiatsu associations to ensure that the curriculum is thorough and includes both theoretical and practical training. Immerse yourself in learning the fundamentals of meridian theory and traditional Chinese medicine, which are the basis of Shiatsu therapy.

You will learn vital skills in hands-on training, including finger pressure, stretches, and joint mobilization, all designed to balance the body's energy flow and support well-being. As you advance, you will work closely with instructors in a clinical setting to hone your abilities and build your self-assurance in providing successful Shiatsu treatments. Finally, you will continue to receive updates on advances in Shiatsu and related fields through workshops and seminars.

After training, obtain certification from reputable Shiatsu organizations to verify your abilities and build credibility. Study hard for certification exams, showcasing your mastery of Shiatsu techniques, anatomy, and ethics. Following certification, further your career by looking for mentorship from experienced practitioners and taking part in continuing education courses. This never-ending learning strategy will enable you to provide customized Shiatsu treatments that successfully address clients' unique health needs.

ESTABLISHING A SHIATSU PRACTICE: SITE AND SUPPLIES

When setting up your Shiatsu practice, it's important to create an environment that makes your clients feel at ease and relaxed. To start, choose a location that embodies the peace that is central to Shiatsu therapy. Look for spaces that have natural lighting, low noise levels, and sufficient ventilation to create a calm atmosphere. Whether you choose to rent a commercial space or set up a home studio, accessibility for clients should come first.

Invest in ergonomic stools or chairs for yourself to maintain proper posture and avoid strain during treatments. Outfit your Shiatsu practice with necessary items like a comfortable massage table or futon, clean linens, and supportive pillows or bolsters to enhance client comfort during sessions. Include relaxing elements like ambient lighting, aromatherapy diffusers with essential oils, and soothing music.

Make sure that your treatment area is well-organized and that supplies like hot/cold therapy packs, massage oils, and hygiene essentials are easily accessible. You should also strictly enforce cleanliness and hygiene standards to maintain professionalism and the trust of your clients. Finally, you should think about implementing technology to manage client records securely, schedule appointments, and accept online bookings to reduce administrative work and improve client convenience.

MARKETING TECHNIQUES TO DRAW CUSTOMERS TO YOUR SHIATSU CLINIC

Craft a compelling brand message that highlights the unique benefits of Shiatsu therapy, emphasizing its ability to promote relaxation, relieve pain, and support overall well-being. This will help you define your target audience based on demographic factors like age, lifestyle, and health concerns. Successful marketing will draw in a steady stream of clients eager to experience the benefits of holistic healing.

Create a polished website that functions as an online storefront for your Shiatsu business. It should have interesting content, client endorsements, and educational blog entries about holistic health issues. You should also optimize your website for search engines to increase online exposure and draw in organic traffic from people looking for alternative healing modalities. Finally, you should strategically use social media platforms to share educational content, client success stories, and live Shiatsu technique demonstrations.

Engage in active networking within your community by attending health fairs, wellness events, and networking groups that are frequented by both healthcare professionals and potential clients.

Work in conjunction with other complementary health practitioners, such as acupuncturists, chiropractors, and yoga instructors, to form referral partnerships and increase the number of new clients you see. Provide introductory sessions or package discounts to entice new clients to try Shiatsu therapy for themselves. Reward them with loyalty programs or seasonal promotions.

STRATEGIES FOR RETAINING CLIENTS AND DEVELOPING A NETWORK OF REFERRALS

Developing a devoted clientele is essential to maintaining a successful Shiatsu business. Concentrate on providing outstanding customer service by creating a friendly atmosphere, paying attention to what clients need, and tailoring treatments to meet their specific health objectives. Create a customized care plan that emphasizes professionalism, empathy, and constant communication to establish rapport and trust with each client.

Encourage regular bookings by implementing client retention strategies like personalized follow-up emails, appointment reminders, and special offers for return visits. Regularly gather feedback through informal conversations or satisfaction surveys to improve service delivery and quickly resolve any issues. Build a positive online reputation by encouraging satisfied customers to leave reviews on websites like Google, Yelp, or social media channels.

Build a strong referral network by fostering relationships with current clients and encouraging them to recommend friends, family, or coworkers who might benefit from Shiatsu therapy. As a thank you for client referrals, consider offering discounted sessions or complimentary add-on treatments. Collaborate with nearby businesses or wellness centers to cross-promote services and broaden your community reach.

BUDGETING AND FINANCIAL ISSUES FOR A SHIATSU PRACTICE

To ensure long-term sustainability, managing the financial aspects of your Shiatsu practice successfully requires careful planning and budgeting. Start by estimating startup costs, which include costs for equipment purchase or rental, training and certification, licensing fees, and initial marketing efforts. Create a thorough business plan that outlines revenue projections, pricing strategies for various services or packages, and expected operating expenses like rent, utilities, and insurance premiums.

Based on market research, competitor analysis, and the value of your specialized skills and expertise, set competitive yet sustainable prices for your Shiatsu sessions. You should also think about providing membership plans or flexible payment options to cater to different client budgets and promote repeat business. Finally, you should put in place effective systems for invoicing and billing that will expedite financial transactions and ensure that you have accurate records for tax purposes.

Track revenue and expenses using accounting software or spreadsheets to keep tabs on your practice's financial performance. Set aside money for continuing education, equipment upkeep, and marketing campaigns to draw in new business and keep hold of current clientele. Create an emergency fund to cover unanticipated costs and changes in client demand to maintain your practice's financial stability during lean times or recessions.

CHAPTER ELEVEN

SHIATSU FAQS AND TROUBLESHOOTING

RESOLVING FREQUENTLY ASKED QUESTIONS ABOUT LEARNING SHIATSU

Understanding the philosophy behind Shiatsu helps newcomers appreciate its therapeutic value, emphasizing harmony and balance within the body. Learning Shiatsu can initially raise questions about its effectiveness and practicality. Beginners often wonder about its benefits compared to other therapeutic methods. Shiatsu stands out for its holistic approach, focusing on the body's energy flow and pressure points to promote relaxation and healing. It doesn't require extensive equipment, making it accessible for both practitioners and clients seeking natural remedies.

FAQs frequently center on the efficacy of Shiatsu for a variety of conditions, such as stress relief, muscle tension, and improving general well-being. By examining these questions, novices can develop confidence in Shiatsu's ability to complement conventional medicine and promote holistic health. Shiatsu practitioners learn to apply gentle pressure along specific meridians to release tension and restore energy flow.

Concerns regarding the learning curve are addressed with practical advice on how, to begin with fundamental techniques and work your way up to more complex ones. Books, online courses, and workshops provide organized learning pathways that guarantee novices gain a firm foundation in Shiatsu principles and techniques. With these common concerns addressed, those new to Shiatsu can set out on their path with clarity and excitement, knowing they are joining a fulfilling field of natural healing.

FAQS REGARDING SHIATSU METHODS AND THEIR USES

When it comes to providing effective therapy, practitioners must understand the various applications of Shiatsu techniques. FAQs frequently focus on the different types of Shiatsu, such as Zen Shiatsu and Namikoshi Shiatsu, which emphasize different approaches to energy balance and therapeutic touch. Newcomers also ask about the specific hand techniques used in Shiatsu, such as finger pressure, thumb kneading, and palm pressure, which are designed to promote relaxation and release tension.

Shiatsu practitioners explain that Shiatsu works by stimulating acupressure points along meridians, encouraging the body's natural healing mechanisms. Answering these questions helps beginners grasp the versatility of Shiatsu in addressing both physical and emotional ailments, enhancing overall well-being through non-invasive techniques. FAQs also cover the benefits of Shiatsu for various conditions, from improving digestion and sleep patterns to alleviating back pain and headaches.

Another common question among newcomers is how Shiatsu is applied in different settings, like clinics, spas, and private practices. FAQs offer valuable information about customizing Shiatsu techniques to meet the needs of specific clients, which promotes a more individualized approach to therapy. By answering these questions, practitioners can enhance their knowledge of Shiatsu's therapeutic potential and better equip themselves to provide individualized treatments that support health and vitality.

SOLVING CLIENT PROBLEMS IN SHIATSU SESSIONS

Shiatsu practitioners learn to communicate effectively with clients, address concerns, and modify techniques as necessary to improve therapeutic outcomes. Common challenges that practitioners may face during troubleshooting client issues during sessions include issues like client discomfort or resistance to specific techniques, which call for sensitivity and adaptability. FAQs frequently center on techniques for calming anxious clients and ensuring a comfortable environment conducive to relaxation and healing.

Managing client expectations about the outcome of Shiatsu therapy is another common challenge. FAQs offer advice on how to explain Shiatsu's holistic nature, emphasizing its role in supporting overall wellness instead of offering quick fixes. Practitioners teach clients about the gradual benefits of regular sessions, fostering a therapeutic relationship that is based on mutual trust and understanding over time.

In addition, FAQs address self-care strategies like regular breaks, meditation, and ongoing professional development to enhance skills and prevent fatigue. By proactively addressing these challenges, practitioners can create a supportive environment that maximizes the benefits of Shiatsu for themselves and their clients.

Troubleshooting also includes practical tips for maintaining practitioner energy and focus during sessions, preventing burnout, and ensuring consistent quality of care.

HOW TO TAKE CARE OF YOURSELF AND AVOID BEING A BURNOUT PRACTITIONER

Shiatsu practitioners emphasize the importance of regular exercise, healthy eating, and adequate sleep to sustain energy levels and resilience in demanding therapeutic roles. FAQs center on practical tips for preventing burnout, including setting boundaries with clients, maintaining a balanced schedule, and incorporating personal wellness practices into daily routines. To maintain physical, emotional, and mental well-being, self-care is crucial for practitioners.

The emotional demands of Shiatsu require practitioners to develop self-awareness and compassion for both themselves and their clients. FAQs discuss stress-reduction tactics, including journaling, relaxation techniques, and reaching out to colleagues via professional associations or supervision. By putting self-care first, practitioners increase their ability to provide effective Shiatsu therapy while maintaining long-term job satisfaction and fulfillment.

FAQs emphasize the importance of attending workshops, continuing education courses, and conferences to stay up to date on advancements in Shiatsu techniques and holistic health practices. Practitioners commit to lifelong learning, fostering a growth mindset that enriches their practice and rekindles their passion for helping others through natural healing modalities. Preventing burnout also involves ongoing professional development and skills enhancement.

RESOURCES FOR CONTINUING EDUCATION AND CAREER DEVELOPMENT

Shiatsu practitioners who want to learn more and advance their careers must have access to resources for continuing education and professional development. FAQs direct practitioners to reliable books, journals, and online courses that cover advanced Shiatsu techniques, meridian theory, and integrative approaches to health and wellness. These resources offer thorough analyses and useful advice for improving therapeutic efficacy and client satisfaction.

FAQs also cover specialization options in Shiatsu, including pediatric, sports, and palliative care, which can be tailored to meet the needs and preferences of a wide range of clients. Practitioners can further enhance their expertise and credibility in the field by enrolling in advanced training workshops and certification programs. Continuing education also helps practitioners maintain high standards of practice and promotes Shiatsu therapy as a profession globally.

Another helpful resource mentioned in FAQs is networking within the Shiatsu community, which promotes cooperation, mentoring, and knowledge sharing among practitioners.

Professional associations and forums provide a forum for practitioners to discuss best practices, exchange experiences, and remain up to date on industry trends and regulatory developments. By participating in these networks, practitioners create a supportive community that furthers their professional development and enriches their journey in Shiatsu therapy.